THE REGENERATIVE REVOLUTION AND NATURAL HEALING

ADVANCED PHYSICAL MEDICINE

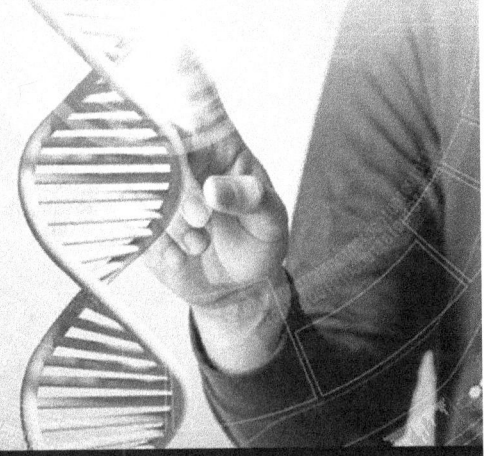

DR. SCOTT HATZENBELER, D.C. & DR. CHRISSY HATZENBELER, D.C.

The Regenerative Revolution and Natural Healing

Helping You Live Life

Dr. Scott Hatzenbeler, D.C.

&

Dr. Chrissy Hatzenbeler, D.C.

The Regenerative Revolution and Natural Healing

Trademark 2021 by Advanced Physical Medicine

All rights reserved. Copyright under Berne Copyright Convention, Universal Copyright Convention, and Pan-American Copyright Convention. No part of this book may be reproduced, stored in a retrieval system, or transmitted in any form, or by any means, electronic, mechanical, photocopying, recording or otherwise, without prior permission of the author.

ISBN: 9798748601450

Published by Advanced Physical Medicine

Disclaimer

While the authors have used their best efforts in preparing this book, they make no representations or warranties with respect to accuracy or completeness of the contents of this book. The advice and strategies contained herein may not be suitable for your situation. You should consult a professional where appropriate. The authors shall not be liable for any loss of profit or any other special, incidental, consequential, or other damages. The purchaser or reader of this publication assumes responsibility for the use of these materials and information. Adherence to all applicable laws and regulations, both advertising and all other aspects of doing business in the United States or any other jurisdiction, is the sole responsibility of the purchaser or reader.

Special Thanks & Dedications

This book is dedicated to our parents; that showed us that through love and perseverance we could accomplish our goals of becoming top doctors in our field. They gave us the support we needed when our goals seemed impossible to achieve and told us to never give up. The success we have experienced has been due to the endless support of many phone calls as well as talks, sometimes even late at night when our dreams seemed too far to reach. Well, here we are, thanks to them.

Table of Contents

TABLE OF CONTENTS	**5**
CHAPTER 1	**7**
Dr. Scott Hatzenbeler, D.C.	7
CHAPTER 2	**10**
Dr. Chrissy Hatzenbeler, D.C.	10
CHAPTER 3	**12**
Regenerative Medicine	12
CHAPTER 4	**19**
Platelet Rich Plasma	19
CHAPTER 5	**24**
Trigger Point Injections	24
CHAPTER 6	**32**
Chiropractic Care	32
CHAPTER 7	**38**
Arm & Shoulder Pain	38
CHAPTER 8	**41**
Carpal Tunnel Syndrome	41
CHAPTER 9	**47**
Digestive Issues	47
CHAPTER 10	**53**
Headaches & Migraines	53
CHAPTER 11	**59**
Intervertebral Disc Problems	59
CHAPTER 12	**65**

Lower Back Pain	65
CHAPTER 13	**68**
Mid Back Pain	68
CHAPTER 14	**72**
Neck Pain	72
CHAPTER 15	**75**
Sciatica Pain	75
CHAPTER 16	**79**
Scoliosis	79
CHAPTER 17	**84**
Rehabilitative Exercises	84
CHAPTER 18	**86**
Motor Vehicle Accidents	86
CHAPTER 19	**92**
Spinal Rehabilitation	92
CHAPTER 20	**97**
Sport Injuries	97
CHAPTER 21	**100**
Durable Medical Equipment	100
CHAPTER 22	**104**
Food and Chemical Sensitivity Testing	104
CHAPTER 23	**108**
Vitamin B12	108

Chapter 1

Dr. Scott Hatzenbeler, D.C.

About Dr. Scott Hatzenbeler D.C

Dr. Scott Hatzenbeler D.C. C.M.V.I or Dr. Scott as all his patient's call him, received his first chiropractic adjustment when he was 21 years old, after being rear-ended at 55 m.p.h. The accident was so violent that the force actually tore his car seat, along with him in it, out of the floorboard of the vehicle. For 4-6 weeks, Dr. Scott suffered from a severe whiplash injury that left him with headaches, visual disturbances, as well as numbness in both hands. Due to the several medications he was put on (pain pills, anti-inflammatories, and muscle relaxers) that were not effective in treating the cause of the problem, Dr. Scott found a local chiropractor. After several months of adjustments to his spine, he was completely back to 100% pre-accident status (no symptoms), due to the cause being corrected, not just the treatment of his symptoms. This is when his goals of going to medical school were drastically outweighed by the overwhelming drive to become a Doctor of Chiropractic instead. Twenty-six years later and thousands of chiropractic adjustments to hundreds of his patients, Dr. Scott Hatzenbeler still has the same compassion for caring for people as he did his very first patient. This attribute of his willingness to serve, his upbeat outlook in life, along with his relentless support to his patients has been some of the many reason's patients seek out his care.

Chapter 2

Dr. Chrissy Hatzenbeler, D.C.

About Dr. Chrissy Hatzenbeler D.C

Dr. Chrissy Hatzenbeler D.C. or Dr. Chrissy, as all her patient's call her, is a third-generation chiropractor. Dr. Chrissy's father (still seeing patients to this day) and her grandfather are both chiropractors, as well as uncles and cousins. All in all, Dr. Chrissy has a total of 7 chiropractors in her family. If anyone truly understands the science and philosophy behind the Chiropractic world, it would be Dr. Chrissy. She has had regular chiropractic adjustments from birth and has never had a major illness that her body has not been able to correct on its own. She lives a healthy lifestyle, and she tries to teach all of her patients to try to live to the best of their comfort level as well. The past 18 years of patient care has made Dr. Chrissy one of the most sought out female chiropractors in the area. Please give Dr. Chrissy a call to begin your journey to a healthier you.

Chapter 3

Regenerative Medicine

What is regenerative medicine?

The body is a powerful thing: constructed with the building blocks needed to help heal itself. But as the body ages, those regenerative abilities slow dramatically, and we are left with the question:

Is there a way to supplement our body's ability to heal itself?

We believe so.

Regenerative medicine is the branch of medicine that creates methods to regrow, repair or replace damaged or diseased cells, organs, or tissues. Regenerative medicine includes the generation and use of therapeutic mesenchymal stem cells, growth factors, growth proteins, hyaluronic acid, and many other cellular tissues all put together. These Human Cellular Tissue Products are most often commonly referred to by the public, as Stem Cell Therapy. When one is born, there is approximately 1 stem cell for every 10,000 cells in your body. By the time you are 80 there is approximately 1 stem cell for every 2 million cells in the body. Even though there are stem cells in our human cellular tissue products, there is much more to this type of procedure than just stem cells. Our products are intentionally derived from two tissue sources: the Wharton's jelly layer of the umbilical cord as well as placental tissue. These rich, potent tissue sources are uniquely able to help protect, cushion and support injured parts of the body as well as aid the optimal regenerative environment. By using human cellular tissue products from the umbilical cord (Wharton's Jelly) of healthy, full term, newborn babies, the patient is given the ability to heal at a much faster rate. But to be effective, you must put in the work. That's why we insist on the best companies to produce the products, as well as, having rigorous research behind every product we use. By going the extra step to identify the optimal tissue source from which we get our human cell and tissue products (HCT/P's), we hope to better support the body's natural regenerative environment, and aid in its repair. The regenerative medicine products we use have years of research behind it, are thoroughly tested, verified by independent parties, and meticulously handled from labs to our medical office. Why? Because our products have a purpose that's bigger than just business: to help heal every*body*. The theory behind these products is to have these specific products regenerate tissues that have been degenerating over the years or to address current trauma that the patient is suffering from. These Human Cellular Tissue Products (HCT/P's) can not only prevent possible surgery but allow the patient to regain the ability to do the things they once were able to do.

How do you treat for this?

We start by putting patients on a high level regenerative 10-day nutritional program to support the soft tissue in the area. This sort of preps, if you will, the tissue around the area of concern to maximize the results for the patient. The patient first starts off with a medical examination to the area of concern followed by the necessary x-rays. The patient's whole body is taken into consideration not just the symptoms. For example: A patient with degenerative knees that have been told they need surgery, or a knee replacement are looked at from the ground up. We would look at their feet for any imbalances, range of motion assessment of the low back, since many people with knee trouble seem to have back concerns as well, orthopedic exam on both knees, and then x-rays to determine if the regenerative medicine is right for them. We have a couple simple rules in our clinic; it must be good for the patient and it must be compliant with all regulatory agencies to proceed. Once the necessity has been determined, the patient is then given the 10-day nutritional products, then they arrive in our office for their motion assessments, and then given the injection of the human cellular tissue products. Many patients also become interested in chiropractic and rehabilitative exercises to enhance the outcome as well. The great news for the patient is that the procedure itself is done in under an hour, performed in-office, and the patient walks out the door and back to their day or work that same day. And there aren't any painful months of rehab and no downtime is needed.

How do patients feel after this treatment?

Patients usually at most, feel a little achy in the joint that has been injected with the human cellular tissue products or feel a "sloshing" around the joint due to the product that has been injected the first day. By the first week, many patients have described a noticeable decrease in pain. By the first month most patients have shown an improvement in their range of motion of that joint along with continued decrease in pain. In the months that follow, patients are typically beginning to do activities that they have not been able to do in a long time with little to no pain at all.

What is the most common question you get asked about that treatment?

Where do these stem cells come from? These cells come from the placenta tissue as well as umbilical cords from full term healthy delivered babies. Both parents must give full consent and take a drug test either 7 days before the birth of the child or 7 days after the birth of the child. The Regenerative medicine is then quarantined for 30 days to test for many other things that do not make the products pure. If strict policies are not upheld, then the tissue sample is discarded.

What question SHOULD someone ask you about this treatment?

What can or what can't they do in their lifestyle after they receive the injections. This is important because the patient needs to take it easy for about 4 weeks following the procedure. The patient can typically follow their activities of daily living if it doesn't create a strain to the area being treated. You don't just want to pick up a golf club and go play golf for the afternoon or hit the gym for a great workout either. Common sense dictates that the patient just move the joint in its normal fashion and take it relatively easy for the first 30 days. Another thing that the patient must do, is to

NOT use any anti-inflammatory medication after the injection. One must take into consideration that a small amount of swelling after the injection is not necessarily a bad situation. You see, when one injures an area of the body, especially a joint, then swelling usually is present and is required by the body to begin the healing process. This is exactly the time when all your healing cells, including stem cells, rush in through this inflammatory response and begin to regenerate tissues that need to be repaired.

What is the biggest misconception about the treatment?

The biggest misconception is that these cells come from aborted babies. This is not only a false statement, but it is illegal to use cells from aborted babies as well. Those cells are known as Embryonic stem cells. The stem cells that are in our products come from, as mentioned previously, from full term delivered healthy babies, in which both parents have given their consent, as well as been drug tested on top of that. The cells that are in our product are known as Mesenchymal stem cells. These cells that come from the umbilical cord known as Wharton's Jelly, are the highest concentration of stem cells found within the human body.

Chapter 4

Platelet Rich Plasma

What is platelet rich plasma?

Better known as PRP, Platelet Rich Plasma is another regenerative medicine procedure that instead of using somebody else's stem cells and growth factors, we use your stem cells along with all your growth factors found naturally in your blood. You typically do not have the amount of stem cells and growth factors as you age compared to a newborn's, but this is a great treatment for people typically under 60 years of age. After the age of 60 you start to take a gamble on the success of the outcome based on the patient's age and not having the amount of healing qualities found within one's own blood.

How do you treat for this?

The patient is brought back for a full consultation with Dillon, our Case Manager who has been highly trained to take time to understand, listen, and ask about every single detail that has created the concern of why the patient is seeking this service. Just because a patient might have heard great things about this procedure, it still must be right for the patient, as well as meet the compliance to begin such a treatment. Once we feel this is a good option for the patient to explore, the patient is personally introduced to our medical provider and begins a full comprehensive exam on the areas of concern. After the exam and appropriate x-rays are performed, the patient is then scheduled for an x-ray review and explanation in detail of their problems and scheduled for the procedure that day. The procedure begins with a simple blood draw from the patient which is then spun in a centrifuge for a certain amount of time to pack the red blood cells to the bottom of the test tube. This leaves the clear liquid on top (plasma), which is where your stem cells and other things like growth hormones and growth factors, among various other things that help repair are found. The plasm is then drawn up and injected into the joint of concern. This is performed every 2 weeks for a total of 3 injections. The patient is also recommended to have typically, a short 4-week plan of therapeutic exercises to strengthen the area as well.

How do patients feel after this treatment?

Typically, the patient may experience some minor discomfort around the injection site with a heavy or dull achy feeling due to the patient's plasma creating a minor "trauma like" situation in the area of concern. This is a good thing because we are trying to create this situation for the body to send certain cells to that area to commence the healing effort. The patient during this phase is told not to use any anti-inflammatories or ice due to this reaction being the exact thing we are looking for. This soreness usually dissipates within a few hours and may be a little sore the next day even. However, the soreness goes away as the body begins its repair stage. The majority of our patients report back to us that with each injection every two weeks comes a little more relief and improved range of motion.

What is the most common question you get asked about this treatment?

The biggest question posed about the treatment is the cost and does insurance cover it? The answer I typically give to this question is, the question right back to them... Do YOU think insurance covers this? It is amazing that the answer I get back a high percentage of the time is... Well, since I have heard so much good about it, then probably no. To which I respond, unfortunately you are correct.

What question SHOULD someone ask you about this treatment?

If I feel a huge improvement after the first or second injection, should I not get the third? The answer here is absolutely continuing. This has been a heavily researched and proven method based on three injections. Not one or two, because it is based on functional results not merely relief of symptoms.

What is the biggest misconception about this treatment?

That getting PRP is similar to getting regenerative medicine, which is not even on the same playing field. Regenerative medicine uses all the stem cells along with many other growth factors mentioned previously from the umbilical cord of healthy newborn babies. PRP is taking all the stems cells and growth factors from your body. The difference is in the age, as well as the number of cells. Think about it, do you typically heal quicker when you're younger or when you're older?

Chapter 5

Trigger Point Injections

What are trigger point injections?

To understand what Trigger Point Injections are, one must first understand what a Trigger Point is. A Trigger Point is a taut band of skeletal muscle that creates a discrete, hyperirritable area or region of the body. They can be painful when pressed upon or can produce referred pain (pain in another region) by traveling along the nerves that are intertwined within the muscle fibers. Anyone can be affected. A recent study shows that approximately 90% of the public have Trigger Points.

How do you treat for this?

One of our team of medical professionals performs the natural Trigger Point Injections. We start by using Lidocaine, a local anesthetic, to simply reduce the pain right from the start, but within the injection is also a homeopathic all-natural solution with plant enzymes that help to break up the adhesions that are found trapped within the muscle fibers. Do you ever feel those "knots" in your shoulders that are hard and most often tender to the touching pressure of one's fingers? Those are the muscles or areas that are injected to break loose the adhesions and help restore the muscle back to the best it can be. After the patient is injected, they are free to go without any major restrictions. The protocol for this treatment is only twice a week for approximately four weeks.

How do patients feel after this treatment?

Each patient has their own feelings after these injections. Some experience a sore achy feeling from the fibers being slightly disrupted, but most patients report a decrease of pain to the area due to the lidocaine. However, as time goes on and the patient has the taut muscle fibers broken down there is a big difference not only in the decrease of pain in that area of the body, but the muscles fibers that have been broken down naturally have better functionality to them as well.

What is the most common question you get asked about this treatment?

Does it hurt? Usually the only pain or discomfort, which is more what we tend to hear about is from the little pinch from the needle itself. The needles themselves are very small and most often the patient reports that they didn't even really notice the injection as it was performed. Most of the discomfort comes from the breaking down of those adhesions from the muscle fibers as the muscle engages in its normal activity. We hear many times from patients that it feels like they received a deep tissue massage in that area.

What question SHOULD your patients ask you about this treatment?

The best question asked about the procedure, in our opinion, is "What is this actually doing for me?" This question shows the provider that the patient is engaged and wanting to know more about the benefits of this fantastic natural approach. At this point the patient is explained in detail to what a Trigger Point is and why it should be broken down. If you have an educated patient, then you have a more compliant patient, which ultimately leads to a better outcome for the patient.

What is the biggest misconception about this treatment?

The biggest misconception we feel the patient has towards the procedure is that needles hurt. As mentioned before, the needles are very small and do NOT outweigh the long-term benefits that this natural solution provides. In fact, we often joke with our patients, stating that we would be more concerned if you told us that you really liked needles and injections.

Do I Have Trigger Points?

Trigger points commonly cause:

- muscle or areas sensitive to pressure
- burning, achy, dull pain
- tight, stiff muscles
- muscle spasms
- pain that travels to the arms or legs
- headaches or migraines
- numbness
- pain that diminishes with heat application

How are Trigger Point Injections (TPI) performed?

The Nurse Practitioner will clean the area to be injected over the trigger point and use a tiny needle to inject through the skin. If you have ever had a TB skin injection, it is even smaller than this needle.

The needle can cause a small "twitch" which tells the nurse the proper placement has been reached. A small amount of numbing medication and Sarapin is then injected. The patient may feel slight burning but quickly disappears.

It is the combination of the needle itself causing the "twitch" and the injected medication that relieves the pain and muscle spasms. There isn't research to support the effects of Sarapin but this medication has been used since the 1930's and the only reported side effects are headache and lightheadedness. The injection overall only takes a couple of minutes, afterwards pressure will be applied and massaged into the muscle with a special device called PTLMS.

What are the results of trigger point injections?

Right away patients typically feel relief as the numbing medication starts acting within a minute. This pain relief will last between 4 and 12 hours, and then it wears off. After the injections some experience soreness, just like a vaccine shot type of healing.

Stretching may help at this point, applying ice to the injected area also helpful. No heating pads for the first 24 hours and keep the area clean and dry. Call your nurse if you experience rash or fever after injections. Adding a TENS unit with intermittent use may aid in pain relief. After the numbing medication wears off, pain relief from the Sarapin should "kick in" and provide additional relief anywhere from a few days to months. Most patients report long lasting relief after the treatment is completed.

Typically trigger point injections are repeated 2 times a week for 4 weeks and are often performed in conjunction with physical rehabilitation (physical therapy type exercises), chiropractic, and massage.

What are the risks of trigger point injections?

The risks of these injections are very low. There is a small risk of infection, bleeding, redness, and allergic reaction to the injectables. Make sure to tell your provider if you are taking a blood thinner such as Aspirin or Coumadin.

There is also an extremely rare incident of the needle inadvertently puncturing the lung or other organ. If the patient develops chest pain, cough, or shortness of breath after the procedure or severe nausea and vomiting, the nurse practitioner should be notified.

Another risk is that the injection may not work. If TPI's are done too frequently scar tissue can form in the area being treated.

At Advanced Physical Medicine our Certified Nurse Practitioner is trained and experienced in this procedure and in all aspects of relieving pain. This often includes trigger point injections along with individualized care plans to achieve the best results for complicated patients.

Chapter 6

Chiropractic Care

What is Chiropractic care?

Chiropractic is an overall way of looking at the human body. It's based on the idea that the body is self-sustaining, self-regenerating, and self-healing. The body is in essence completely controlled by the brain through its connection via the spinal cord and the vast networks of nerves that make up the body. When this system is not functioning at its peak, the overall performance of the human body is lacking. In the chiropractic world, drugs and medicine are not utilized as a form of treating a patient. While supplementation and nutrition are almost always a part of the bigger picture, drugs and prescriptions can be viewed as band-aids to treat symptoms rather than going to the source and treating the real problem. This is why we see such great results from regenerative medicine. We must always remember that we should be always asking, why does my knee, shoulder, hip, even need regenerative medicine to begin with. Chiropractic addresses the biomechanics that may have been at the root cause of the whole problem to begin with. We find very often that our patients that get some chiropractic/ rehabilitative care along with the regenerative medicine have much more improved results.

How do you treat for this?

First, the patient is brought into a private room with our case manager to go over every detail that is a concern to the patient. After that, the patient is introduced to our medical provider and all the concerns are then repeated, in front of the patient, to make sure that nothing is missed so that the provider and patient are on the same page. An examination along with the necessary x-rays are then taken. The patient is put on a few passive therapies such as electronic muscle stimulation to reduce the pain in the specific region and/or mechanical traction to stretch the spine out to release some tension in the area of concern. The patient is then scheduled to come back for their report of findings, where everything is one-on-one explained to the patient about what we have found, and recommendations given to what needs to be done. Once the patient has a firm understanding of their issues and how we can help, the patient is again given some passive therapies and begins to receive their chiropractic adjustments.

How do patients feel after this treatment?

Following the patient's adjustment most often, the patient immediately feels some degree of relief. A sense of relaxation is another response that we hear as well.

What is the most common question you get asked about this treatment?

More than a question about the adjustment, is the concern about if the adjustment will hurt. Some patients have the fear of their neck being "cracked", while other patients unfortunately, have been told by other types of doctors how ineffective they feel Chiropractic care is. Even though you can educate the patient on the fallacy of Chiropractic being ineffective and the bias of non-educated providers that do not hold a doctorate degree in the field of Chiropractic, one still may have the fear of being adjusted. This is where our methods put most of those concerns to bed. At Advanced Physical Medicine, we use one of the most advanced technologies in our industry known as the Pro-Adjuster. This is one of the world's first computerized methods of adjusting the spine or most any joint in the body. Yes, the adjustment is performed by a computer. The computer first takes a reading of the amount of stiffness found throughout the spine through the use of a special handheld device using a sensor attached to it called a piezoelectric sensor. Not only does the computer analyze the stiffness in the area of complaint, but also it uses the hand help instrument to gently apply percussive motions to the spine until the area of stiffness has been reduced. In essence, the computer is constantly analyzing and adjusting the joints in real time and listening to the body's tissue response to know when to stop. This in turn reduces the amount of pressure that is on the nerve and therefore reduces or completely eliminates the pain.

What question SHOULD patients ask you about this treatment?

We love when patients want to hear more about the instrument. This is showing us that the fear of being adjusted is beginning to disappear and the confidence to begin care or continue on is being addressed for the patient. Again, if you have an educated patient on your procedures and practices, then you have a more compliant patient, which leads most often to the patient achieving the results they desire. So, some of the best questions we get asked, is about how this instrument actually works.

What is the biggest misconception about this treatment?

We often ask patients in their initial consultation, "What have you heard about Chiropractic care both positive or negative?" The answers we mostly hear are good things about Chiropractic care, but sometimes we run into one of the most common answers which is, "I hear once you start care you always have to go. There is never an end." We immediately explain to the patient that this is absolutely not true at all. However, we do have hundreds of patients that return for additional care after their treatment recommendations are complete. Many patients return for regular adjustments to maintain the correction they have achieved, but that is solely up to the patient and is never required. Think of it like changing the oil in your car. If it isn't making a sound or is performing just right, are you never going to change the oil again? And since you went to the dentist to get a teeth cleaning, are you to never brush your teeth again? Our patients have a definite starting date as well as a definite stopping date for services recommended in our office.

Chapter 7

Arm & Shoulder Pain

Arm & Shoulder Pain

Arms are usually a very flexible part of the body, yet when they start malfunctioning, a person does experience many other problems as well. Dealing with shoulder or arm pain might seem rather simple, but in fact this is certainly not so. One wrong move and it could easily render the limbs immobile. At Advanced Physical Medicine, we are one of the best and most advanced chiropractic clinics, offering clients the best of the best in all regards.

Contrary to popular belief shoulder, arm, or even hand pain is exceptionally common, and many issues of this nature are likely to be linked to a group of nerves, known as the brachial plexus. The said nerves run from the lower neck region through the upper shoulder area and consequently allow the shoulder and arms to move and feel various sensations. The most prominent symptoms which point to this problem include-

- Numbness in the region of the shoulder, arms and even hands
- Intense shoulder ache
- Tingling or uncomfortable burning sensation
- Weakness in the shoulder or arm region.

If you experience any of the above, rather than stressing out or being scared- it is imperative to visit a doctor as soon as possible. Rather than trusting just any and every one for the job. Opting for chiropractic treatment is a safe and effective way to nip the problem in the bud when it has just begun or even to manage it when things have become too unbearable to treat it. Unlike many in the business who make tall claims, Advanced Physical Medicine can provide top of the line treatment at exceptionally affordable prices. Once you try us, you will come to know how well we do our job and how we have truly carved a niche for ourselves in terms of the physical medicine model.

In this regard our chiropractic treatment and therapy procedure will begin with a thorough examination of the patient. This examination will enable the chiropractor to state beyond a shadow of a doubt where the problem is emanating from and what is causing the compression of the nerves. So, if you have been on the lookout for a safe and effective treatment for the problem, chiropractic care is the way to go. Place your trust in us but once and we will certainly not disappoint.

Chapter 8

Carpal Tunnel Syndrome

Chiropractic Treatment for Carpal Tunnel Syndrome

When you experience weakness, numbness, tingling or burning pain in your wrists and parts of your hand, you might want to ask your doctor to check for carpal tunnel syndrome. The carpal tunnel is basically a small and narrow passage in the wrist. The median nerve which extends through the length of the arm moves into the carpal tunnel. It controls the feeling and movement of all your fingers except the pinky. The median nerve is compressed when there is a swelling in the carpal tunnel. This causes the Carpal Tunnel Syndrome (CTS).

What Causes Carpal Tunnel Syndrome?

Excessive pressure on your median nerve or your wrist can cause pain in the carpal tunnel. Obstructed blood flow is one of the main reasons that cause inflammation in the wrist. There are many conditions that can lead to carpal tunnel syndrome and some of the most common among them are;

- High blood pressure
- Pregnancy
- Diabetes
- Menopause

- Rheumatoid arthritis
- Wrist fractures

However, repeated extension of the wrist can also cause inflammation of the median nerve and it can lead to carpal tunnel syndrome. Some of the other causes for CTS are;

- Overextending your wrist for repeated motions such as playing the piano or typing
- Over usage of handheld power tools
- Placing your wrist in an extended manner while using the keyboard

CTS – Who Are At Risk of Developing It?

Carpal Tunnel Syndrome is likely to affect women more than men maybe because women have smaller carpal tunnel. However, it can affect anyone, and it is often diagnosed between 30 and 60 years. People who are employed in certain occupations such as construction work, manufacturing and so forth are at a greater risk of developing this syndrome.

CTS – Symptoms

One of the most frequent symptoms that you might notice is pain in the wrist that might interfere with your sleep. Numbness and pain on the first three fingers of your hand and thumb is another symptom of CTS. You might also drop objects and feel that your hand has "fallen asleep". Symptoms also include a burning pain that travels up your arm.

CTS – Diagnosis

It is quite difficult to identify the underlying cause of Carpal Tunnel Syndrome and diagnosis can be quite perplexing. In some cases, patients may suffer from other medical conditions which exhibit similar symptoms and can be misdiagnosed. Doctors use a combination of physical examinations and tests to diagnose this syndrome. Diagnosis also includes nerve conduction studies which assess the speed of your nerve impulses. If these impulses are slow and abnormal, then you might have CTS.

CTS – Treatment

Carpal Tunnel Syndrome Treatment often depends on the severity of pain and other symptoms. Invasive treatments such as surgery and steroids are often unsuccessful and therefore it is less recommended.

Chiropractic Methods of Treatment

We, at Advanced Physical Medicine, recommend non-invasive chiropractic methods of treatment for CTS. More than often the healing power of chiropractic is seldom taken into consideration. However, it is one of the most powerful alternative treatments for Carpal Tunnel Syndrome. Our chiropractors are trained to investigate and identify the cause of nerve compressions. Our chiropractic methods of treatment involve non-invasive procedures that rely on the natural ability of the body to recuperate.

Carpal Tunnel Syndrome is not an ailment that must be overlooked as it can cause permanent muscle damage and possible loss of functions of your hand. So it is wise to prevent an unnecessary surgery by quickly consulting one of our chiropractors if you think you have CTS.

How Can You Avoid Carpal Tunnel Syndrome?

There are many ways to prevent and reduce the risk of developing CTS. Lifestyle changes and timely treatment of arthritis, high blood pressure and diabetes can help to prevent carpal tunnel syndrome. You must also avoid activities that overexert your wrists to reduce symptoms.

Chapter 9

Digestive Issues

Digestive issues

Blame it on your diet, sedentary lifestyle or inactivity, digestive issues have become a constant nagging problem in almost every person's life. When digestion slows down due to many reasons, it causes severe problems. It can affect your physical and mental well-being. At Advanced Physical Medicine we have had great success helping people regain proper bowel function.

What are Digestive Issues?

Symptoms and causes of digestive disorders vary from one person to another. However, the most common digestive issues are Irritable Bowel Syndrome, Constipation, Chronic Heartburn, Diarrhea, Crohn's disease and so forth. No matter what type of digestive disorders you may have, symptoms range from abdominal pain, bloating, gas, belching flatulence to changes in bowel habits. You may have one or more of these symptoms when you have a digestive disorder.

Digestive problems are often caused due to food allergies, sensitivities, and food intolerances. Today there are a large number of tests which can be done to identify the cause of indigestion. One test that is of importance is called the Alcat Food Sensitivity test. This is a simple blood draw from our medical provider who then ships your blood overnight to a special laboratory that exposes your blood to over 180 different foods, outdoor pollutants, medications, grasses, molds, etc. to see if your blood reacts to any of the tested items to your blood. Then a special in-depth report is sent to our provider who then sits down with you to go over the results that food may have on your body, that could be causing some or all your digestive issues.

How can Digestive Disorder be cured?

Digestive disorders can be quite problematic and can affect the daily life of a person. It can cause serious impediments in food consumption too. As there are so many symptoms pertaining to digestive ailments such as acid reflux, gut leak, lactose intolerance, heartburn and abdominal pain, medical treatment may also vary accordingly. Surgery is often recommended in some extreme cases when medications fail to alleviate symptoms and bring relief. Nevertheless, it is important to change your dietary lifestyle in order to reduce these symptoms. Dietary changes can minimize symptoms to a great extent, not cure them completely.

Today there are a wide number of medications which can be used to reduce the symptoms caused by digestive disorders. While most of the drugs provide immediate relief and eliminate symptoms, it hardly treats the underlying causes of the issue. In this way, you are caught in a vicious cycle of treatments and digestive disorders without cure.

Chiropractic Treatment for Digestive Disorders

One of the most effective ways to treat digestive issues is with chiropractic treatment. It might seem hard to believe, but the entire digestive system is linked to the nervous system of the body. The nervous system of your body can control various aspects of the digestive tract and its functions. Chiropractic treatment is known to reduce inflammation and expedite the healing process of the body.

We, at Advanced Physical Medicine, highly recommend chiropractic care for all types of digestive disorders as we know that it helps to cure your ailment in a more effective manner. When your spine is misaligned, it stresses the nerves which control the digestive organs, and this can cause chronic acid reflux, heartburn, constipation and irritable bowel syndrome.

As experienced chiropractors we can restore proper motion back to your spine through effective gentle adjustments. As mentioned in chapter 6 we use computers to gently adjust your vertebrae back into proper motion, thus allowing your body to place the vertebrae back to as close of a normal position as possible. This will eliminate the strain on your nerves and allow the digestive system to function appropriately.

Here at Advanced Physical Medicine in Gilbert Arizona we offer one of the best natural treatments for digestive disorders. Our chiropractic treatment is quite different from the traditional methods, as we have a highly skilled team of chiropractors who use gentle and accurate techniques to align the spine, as mentioned before, through the use of computers. Our doctors are experts in identifying and locating improper placement of the vertebrae and correction of subluxations. This technique enables the body to return to its original alignment.

We use this computer assisted adjustment techniques to align the spinal column and use different types of supports such as braces, straps, and tapes as part of the treatment. All of our medical providers have a different approach towards all kinds of ailments and provide natural and non-invasive treatment to help.

We have been providing treatment for digestive disorders for many years now. So, contact us for more information on Chiropractic care for digestive disorders.

Chapter 10

Headaches & Migraines

Headaches and Migraines

In case you think you are the only one suffering from headaches time and again, you are not alone. 9 out of 10 Americans suffer from the same on a daily basis. Some headaches may be dull and cause throbbing pain whereas the other may cause excruciating pain and nausea. Many of those who suffer from constant headaches turn towards medication for pain relief. What they are not aware of is that there are better alternatives for headache relief. At Advanced Physical Medicine we have helped endless amounts of patients with headaches that have tried nearly everything before giving us a try. Most of our patients have been completely satisfied with the outcomes that they have experienced.

The most common headache triggers are:
- Muscle tension in the neck or back
- Bad posture
- Food sensitivity
- Environmental factors (noises, lights, stress)
- Physical behaviors (insomnia, excessive exercise, blood sugar changes)
- Teeth clenching
- Anxiety/Depression

We render some of the most effective chiropractic treatment for tension-type headaches, especially those which originate from the neck. Research studies have proven that chiropractic adjustments provide the most immediate response and relief. Moreover, the chiropractic practices at Advanced Physical Medicine have far fewer side effects and much more long-lasting relief than the prescription drugs.

Also, scientists, as well as researchers, have proven that spinal adjustments will leave no stone unturned for easing out the pain in the back and neck by combining adjustments, massage, exercise, and physical therapy. The techniques we use are designed in such a way that it helps relieve pressure on the joints, reduce inflammation and work ahead for improving the nerve function. Just to let you know that when your body is adjusted and aligned in a proper way, tension all throughout the body can disappear. Having your body in a relaxed state is a prerequisite for proper headache relief.

Moreover, conservative, and drug-free treatments can even reduce not only the severity but also the frequency of migraine headaches. Individuals who are experiencing headaches regularly must maintain a headache diary so that one can deduce the probable factors which may be responsible for causing headaches. If you are the one who is regularly feeling a stab in your back or neck, contact Advanced Physical Medicine in Gilbert, Arizona today. Personalized attention is guaranteed because treatment is according to individual symptoms.

The Headache Solution is the start to a better life.
Sphenopalatine Ganglion Block (SPG):

Headaches are a significant source of stress and pain for many people, they affect over 11% of the American population and cost $2.4 billion each year in health care dollars and lost productivity. There are many existing therapies available, including medication, massage, or invasive therapies like occipital nerve blocks, but usually these therapies simply help with the existing pain, but do not prevent them from occurring or really stop the cause.

A new, innovative therapy is now available and offered at Advanced Physical Medicine called the Sphenopalatine Ganglion Block (SPG). The sphenopalatine ganglion which is a bundle of nerves sits in the back of your nasal bones.

Through a newly developed, needle-less, intranasal infusion technique, we are now capable of blocking these nerves which have been shown to be the cause of multiple forms of headaches including tension headaches, cluster headaches, migraine headaches, atypical headaches, etc. The procedure includes inserting a plastic applicator device into each nostril that allows us to specifically target these nerves, and gently spray the posterior portion of the nasal cavity. A procedure that takes literally 10 seconds! Not only is this procedure fast and needle-less, but it is incredibly effective, and the results are typically felt in less than 90 seconds. Imagine being virtually pain free in seconds!

This treatment option is done over a series of 12 visits, but noticeable results will occur with just the first nasal infusion. The 12 visits allow the appropriate time to desensitize these nerves and prevent headaches from occurring in the future. A few cases will need maintenance therapy which includes one treatment every three or four months (after completion of the initial series). This treatment option is incredibly new, but has been studied repeatedly, and is safe, effective, and fast.

It is projected that this treatment option will change the way that headaches are treated around the world. Currently, it is only being offered in a few clinics, and our Nurse Practitioner has had hands-on training with this procedure. Imagine a life without headaches! Schedule an appointment with our Nurse Practitioner to learn more and see if this option is right for you.

Chapter 11

Intervertebral Disc Problems

Intervertebral Disc Problems

Intervertebral discs are positioned between the vertebrae in the spine. The outside of a disc is made from cartilage, and in the center is a jelly like solution. These discs serve many purposes, including allowing movement of the spine, creating space between the vertebrae, and acting as shock absorbers. The gelatinous middle allows the disc to compress and expand based on impact and movement. At Advanced Physical Medicine, we have many years at aligning intervertebral disc problems.

Trauma to the spine can cause the discs to herniate, bulge, become displaced (slipped disc), or even rupture. Trauma or direct injury to the area is not the only cause, however. As we get older, the discs can begin to weaken and dehydrate.

These conditions can put pressure on the nerves around the spine and cause pain.

If you suffer from one of these injuries, you should see a chiropractor. Surgery is risky, expensive, and requires recovery time. In many cases, you can experience relief from these conditions through gentle chiropractic adjustments, physical rehabilitation, and bracing. By properly aligning the spine, pressure can be relieved on nerves and on the discs themselves. This will reduce and hopefully eliminate your pain and discomfort and allow you to live a normal lifestyle.

How Chiropractic Care Can Help Treat Disc Problems?

As mentioned previously, the spinal disc is a spongy and sensitive pad that is found in between the vertebrae of the spinal column. These discs act as shock absorbers of the spine and hold it in place in the center of the body. When the normal aging process begins, these spinal discs which were filled with fluid begin to harden. As we reach adulthood, the soft material or the discs harden. This is exactly the reason why adults are prone to disc injuries.

What is Disc Herniation or Slip Disc?

Spinal discs are set in between the special bones called vertebrae and the ligaments which connect the bones hold these discs in place. There is hardly any space for the disc to slip. However, when a fluid emerges through a crack in the exterior, it can cause the disc to slip. This is also known as disc herniation. It can cause pain and numbness if it affects the nerves.

There are basically two types of herniated discs-prolapses and protrusions. A prolapsed disc is one that is separated from the rest of the disc as it has over protruded. A protruded disc is one that pushes out of shape.

If the disc pressurizes the spinal cord or the nerves, it can be quite painful. People who suffer from slip discs find it extremely painful to accomplish daily chores such as walking, sitting, sneezing, coughing and so forth.

What are the Symptoms of Disc Problems?
Foot and leg pain:

If you have a herniated disc in your lower back, you could experience intense pain in your buttocks, thigh, and foot. However, if you have a slip disc near your neck, you could experience intense pain on your shoulders, arms, and hands. You may also experience weakness in certain parts of your body where the nerves affect the muscles. It may impair your ability to hold things properly. Herniated discs also cause numbness in some parts of the body which are served by the affected nerves. The symptoms of herniated discs vary according to the position of the injured disc. Although there are many treatments that help to ease the pain, most people prefer to choose chiropractic treatment for disc problems.

Chiropractic Treatment for Disc Problems

The Chiropractic doctors at Advanced Physical Medicine help to treat disc problems effectively. We assure you that chiropractic treatment is one of the safest treatment methods to alleviate the pain and discomfort associated with disc problems.

We will conduct an initial examination, check your medical history and conduct a physical test. This will be followed by neurological and orthopedic tests. In some cases, we may suggest an MRI to assess the problem in depth and then prescribe a suitable treatment plan.

At Advanced Physical Medicine, we have the best medical providers to assist you with your disc problems. We have years of experience in locating and analyzing physical ailments through a series of tests conducted by our specialized team. Our chiropractors are top notch and our physical medicine treatment methods we use follow a holistic healing approach.

We follow a standard routine and secure the required information pertaining to your disc problems. We utilize a comprehensive report of your medical history that includes digital images, X-rays, MRI scans and so forth. This will assist our doctors to analyze the type of disc problem and choose a therapy accordingly. Chiropractic treatments involve gentle adjusting techniques through the use of computers to introduce normal motion back to the spine.

Our efficient team of medical providers also suggests lifestyle changes, nutrition, exercises, and overall wellness concept. When you experience any of the symptoms mentioned in this book that include numbness, pain or weakness in your spine or other related areas, please give us a call and consult with one of our medical providers.

Chapter 12

Lower Back Pain

Lower Back Pain

Physical medicine is safer and often more effective than surgery. Many of the pain-sensing nerves of the spine are in facet joints, the two interlocking "fingers" at the back of each spinal bone. The normally smooth surfaces on which these joints glide, can become rough, irritated, and inflamed.

Surgical treatment often involves removing these facet joints, exposing the spinal cord. Another cause of lower back pain can be a bulging disc putting pressure on the spinal cord or a nearby nerve root. The result is often numbness, tingling, or pain down the leg. Cutting away the bulging disc tissue can permanently alter its ability to separate and cushion the adjacent bones. This rarely addresses the underlying structural causes(s) of the problem.

The physical medicine approach is to help restore and more normal motion and position of affected spinal bones with specific chiropractic adjustments and rehabilitative exercises. The simplicity and success of this approach has been documented in numerous research projects and has helped many patients avoid risky surgery.

Loss of work and untold suffering.

Lower back pain results in millions of dollars of lost work and untold suffering every day. Many factors can be responsible for lower back pain. Improper sitting or lifting, overexertion, trauma, or inherited spinal abnormalities may contribute to the cause.

Chapter 13

Mid Back Pain

Mid Back Pain

When most people the world over think of chiropractors, the first thing which comes to their mind is lower back treatment. Though this is indeed true because over 31 million North Americans do suffer with severe lower back pains, yet mid back pain is indeed something just as common, often known to even exacerbate, lower back pains significantly. Advanced Physical Medicine in Gilbert, Arizona can help in dealing with these issues by using a multi-faceted approach between spinal rehab, gentle spinal adjustments, as well as bracing and injections to help reduce spasms that are often associated with these types of problems.

Finding out the root of the problem is the first step

There can truly be several reasons why you may be experiencing such pains in the mid back region, so rather than ignoring it; it is always a much better option to pay us a visit and avail of help immediately. In such a case, the first thing we will do is attempt to find the root of the problem. Most often it is due to sitting at the computer for long hours that causes this issue. However, in some cases, the pain is likely to be associated with a referred pain or rather a complication from the organs in the region. Some of the most common causes of mid back pain include- lung condition, heart condition, kidney infection etc. This is usually found out by simple exercises or tests.

The main way in which we help in solving this issue, is by doing spinal rehabilitation and gentle spinal adjustments along with any regenerative therapy necessary. Patients who have committed to our services, have been exceptionally happy with the results. Conventionally a misalignment of the spine or other kind of soft tissue can irritate the nervous system significantly. The adjustment, thereby helps in the proper alignment of the spine, thereby eliminating pain and permitting the proper functioning of the nervous system. Any tissue that has been damaged or has been degenerating can also benefit by regenerative medicine as well.

Other methods we make use of include- electrical stimulation as well as ultrasound. It is essential to note that mid back pain is something we can easily deal with at Advanced Physical Medicine, but it might indeed require more than one session. Unlike many other facilities which provide incomplete treatment, we make it a point to provide our patients the best of the best when it comes to both patient care as well as bedside manner. It is certainly not for nothing that we have been able to carve such a considerable niche for ourselves in the competitive chiropractic world.

Chapter 14

Neck Pain

Neck Pain

The Cervical spine, muscles, and nerve tissues surrounding your neck may be affected by several degenerative issues, injuries, or postural problems. It's no wonder that most of the individuals turn towards pain relief drugs and medications totally overlooking the very fact that these are not the only treatments available for obtaining relief.

The cervical spine forms the most fragile and vulnerable part of the vertebral column although the neck always bears the weight of the head. The most common neck injuries include whiplash and auto accident injuries. Sharp and sudden motions can often dislocate the facet joints which articulate with the cervical vertebrae. This also renders normal joint muscle impossible.

Whatever be the underlying cause of your neck pain, you must never go for any kind of risky major surgery. Drugs, no doubt, can provide you temporary relief but they have their own side effects too. Our licensed medical providers at Advanced Physical Medicine, will provide you the best and the most personalized treatment for neck pain, by addressing the underlying reason. We will fail no chance at identifying any vertebrae or disc abnormalities and will administer targeted chiropractic adjustments in order to normalize the cervical alignment, relieving muscle strain as well as resolving joint stiffness.

Always bear in mind that depending upon the neck pain manifested, our team of medical providers at Advanced Physical Medicine might recommend multiple types of treatment. For example, spinal rehabilitation may help treat bulging or herniated discs in the neck, whereas regenerative medicine may reduce inflammation in injured neck muscles. Moreover, therapeutic exercises work ahead by restoring neck function and strength. The experienced providers may even offer personalized counselling on lifestyle as well as postural changes for keeping the neck of the patients in a healthy state.

You must remember that your natural neck pain treatment begins with an appropriate evaluation. Schedule your appointment today and feel the difference.

Chapter 15

Sciatica Pain

Sciatica Pain

Often considered as a promising form of alternative medicine, Chiropractic, mostly pertains to the diagnosis or the treatment of various mechanical ailments or disorders of the musculoskeletal system. Providing chiropractic services are certainly not easy, but it does go a long way in easing the pain and discomfort of the patient. Chiropractic treatment is the preferred course for many when dealing with the issue of Sciatica.

Conventionally caused by the compression of the sensitive sciatica nerve, Sciatica is truly very painful indeed and if not treated in a proper manner can lead to serious consequences. Disorders which are known to bring on the problem include the following-

- Misaligned vertebrae body or bodies
- A slipped disc
- Phenomenon of Childbirth
- Pregnancy
- Tumors

Apart from this it can be brought on by non-spinal disorders as well such as constipation, diabetes or even when people constantly sit on their wallets. In the event of suffering with this problem trusting the best chiropractic treatment provider is the best thing that anyone can really do. At Advanced Physical Medical we offer exemplary physical medicine treatment, that is why people from all over Gilbert, Arizona, and other places as well, seek out our services the moment they are in trouble. We truly stand head and shoulders above the rest in terms of the care we give, we treat sciatica by:

Cold therapy

This numbs the area and reduces inflammation; cold therapy is truly an effective treatment.

Adjustments

Spinal adjustments continue to be one of the most effective ways to handle the situation. It truly is the core of chiropractic care and helps in the reduction of the nerve irritability, which serves as the root of the problem. This method is safe as well as effective.

Trigger Point injections

These are designed to enhance the function of the muscles surrounding the spine. When this method is used in combination with the spinal adjustments and rehabilitative exercises, we often see a much-improved outcome for the patient.

Dealing with sciatica can be hard but getting the proper treatment from a reputable clinic like ours is certainly a step in the right direction.

Chapter 16

Scoliosis

Scoliosis – Causes and Chiropractic Treatment

Although spines appear curved from the sides, it must appear straight when we glance from the front. When the spine is abnormally curved it is known as Scoliosis. Curvature of the spine is one of the most common symptoms of this ailment. There are various types of scoliosis which vary according to the age and the causes of the disorder.

Scoliosis is a complex disease and even experts are unaware of the underlying causes of this ailment. Moreover, there is no proven cure for Scoliosis. However, it is possible to reduce the symptoms of this disease and treat it effectively with medical intervention.

What are the Causes of Scoliosis?

Degenerative scoliosis:

This type of scoliosis occurs in adults due to changes in the structure of the spine. This is mainly caused due to spondylosis. Osteoporosis also affects the spine and can cause abnormal curves in the spine.

Birth defects:

In some cases, the bones of the spine fail to complete each other or separate from one another during the development of the fetus. In such conditions, children develop a C shaped spine, and it is known as congenital. It is one of the most severe forms of scoliosis and it requires treatment.

Muscle spasms

Functional problems such as muscle spasms and other developmental problems can also cause scoliosis. In this case, the spine is normal but other defects in the body can cause an abnormal curve in the spine.

Treatment for Scoliosis

Treatment for scoliosis is based on the severity of the disease or the curve. It is also determined according to type of scoliosis. Bracing and surgery are the two types of treatments that are usually prescribed for people suffering from scoliosis.

Chiropractic treatments are more effective in treating scoliosis. At Advanced Physical Medicine, we recommend chiropractic treatment along with exercise, natural medical approaches, and bracing for scoliosis because it helps to relieve the symptoms in a more effective manner.

Chiropractic Treatment Based on the Type of Scoliosis

Unlike the traditional chiropractic methods, we provide specific treatment for scoliosis based on the type of the ailment. We can achieve this because of working together with our medical providers to give more of a whole-body approach. We aim to gradually correct the spine using techniques that are gentle and accurate. Our treatments are beneficial to people of all ages and medical conditions.

Although most people believe that a sideway curve in the spine is termed as scoliosis, the truth is the ailment is much more complex than that. There are three natural curves in the spine and due to scoliosis, the spine is forced in a different direction.

People suffering from scoliosis have unstable joints and risk dislocations and injuries if they are not treated properly. We use specific and precise mechanical instruments which are used to adjust the structure of the spine, neck and other joints in the body.

Re-centering the head is the first step involved in the chiropractic treatment for scoliosis. Precise and gentle adjustment instruments are used to massage the neck into its ideal position. Several other adjustment treatments are also performed on the hips and other joints of the body according to the X-ray results.

There are a number of chiropractors who provide specialized treatments for scoliosis. However, it is important to choose the best chiropractors as the treatment must be given by an experienced practitioner.

Is Scoliosis Curable and Preventable?

For the present, there is no cure for scoliosis apart from the effective treatments mentioned above. As surgery is unlikely to solve the problem, most people opt for non-invasive treatments which are more effective. There is no way to prevent scoliosis as the causes for this ailment is quite unclear. Doctors believe that certain exercises and yoga can aggravate scoliosis as it involves twisting the spine. Nevertheless, symptoms of scoliosis can be reduced to a great extent with chiropractic treatments.

Chapter 17

Rehabilitative Exercises

What are rehabilitative exercises?

Advanced Physical Medicine has Spinal Rehab Technicians performing Spinal Rehabilitation. The restoration of spinal form and function is a complicated process. It is not just one protocol for temporary symptom relief, but a systems approach to achieve a long-term and positive result. Injuries and/or displacements of the spine require special treatment and in the proper sequence to restore the spine's form and function. The role of water intake, supplements, warm-up stretching exercises, force-over-time traction, and isometric-demand exercises, as well as the use of controlled vibration in modern treatment, cannot be refuted. Individual therapies used by themselves are of little benefit in restoration of spinal soft- and hard-tissue form and function in the spinal screw matrix closed kinetic system. Therefore, understanding and using proven protocols of therapeutic exercises is appealing.

Chapter 18

Motor Vehicle Accidents

What are the Benefits of Physical Medicine Care After A Motor Vehicle Accident?

Physical medicine care is one of the best alternative medical treatments after a motor vehicle accident as it hardly involves surgery or medications. We recommend chiropractic treatment, as well as rehab and trigger point injections after an accident due to many reasons. People with minor injuries hardly consider visiting a chiropractor as most of them are unaware of the amazing benefits.

Why Visit A Physical Medicine Clinic After A Motor Vehicle Crash?

Non-invasive treatment is the number one goal, that's why.

Physical medicine care is the best alternative to surgery as the treatment involves realigning the spine and joints which help to reduce pain and inflammation. There is hardly any need for surgery when natural treatment immediately after an accident is given a chance first. However, there is a large percentage of people that actually require surgery after an accident. Our job is to exhaust every option for you naturally first before going through those steps in that direction.

Minimizes inflammation

In some cases, there may be micro tears in your muscles or ligaments which can cause severe pain after an accident. These tears are seldom visible in X-rays and it is difficult to diagnose. We are highly trained to realign the spine and reduce pain and inflammation in the body by receiving the pressure on the nerves in the area of complaint and the surrounding tissues that support that area.

Relief from pain without drugs

Pain relief medications cease the pain and offer relief for a short period of time. It seldom heals the damage caused by the accident. In due course of time, it is possible to become addicted to these medications and it may also cause withdrawal symptoms when it is stopped abruptly. Chiropractic along with natural medical care helps to reduce pain by addressing the source of the pain. It heals the actual injury instead of reducing or eliminating pain for a short period of time.

Invisible injuries

Some injuries such as whiplash are less obvious, and it can be quite painful. Symptoms of whiplash may appear only after a while, which include dizziness, numbness, and nagging pain. Even if you tend to ignore the symptoms and pain for a short time, it might worsen and aggravate your problems. So, it is wise to consult a physical medicine office after a motor vehicle accident to seek treatment for pain and inflammation. A highly trained medical provider can diagnose injuries and initiate treatment before the pain becomes intolerable.

Mobilizes your body

Inflammations caused due to back or neck injuries can be quite troublesome, and it can affect the healing power of your body. Chiropractors adjust your neck and spine through therapies to mobilize your spine. It will also help to restore the mobility of your body and expedite the healing process. Here at Advanced Physical Medicine, we are trained and hold certifications to specifically offer specialized treatment to accident victims.

Spinal Adjustments

Another benefit of visiting a physical medicine office after a motor vehicle injury is that chiropractic treatments involve spinal adjustments along with exercises that help to release hormones which reduce pain. These hormones help in healing the body and reducing inflammation caused due to injuries sustained from a car crash.

Scar tissues

After a motor vehicle accident scar tissues tend to develop on the muscles which can be quite painful and worrisome. Through trigger point injections, as mentioned in previous chapters, these scar tissues break up easily and let the body heal on its own at a quicker pace. An expert medical provider can identify scar tissues and focus on healing the injured area of your body.

No long term pain

When there are no visible injuries, most people refrain from visiting doctors. This can prove to be detrimental in the future as minor and invisible injuries can aggravate. It is important to consult with our office, or a physical medicine office, near you immediately after a car crash as it will prevent long term problems from arising. A physical medicine team approach can identify, diagnose, and treat a medical condition before it aggravates into a serious ailment.

Therefore, it is important to consult an office like ours and receive treatment if you were injured or hurt in a motor vehicle accident. Advanced Physical Medicine has been providing assistance to accident victims for many decades now. We have the required training and expertise to help you overcome pain through natural methods of healing.

Chapter 19

Spinal Rehabilitation

Spinal Rehabilitation

The restoration of spinal form and function is a complicated process. It is not just one protocol for temporary symptom relief, but a systems approach to achieve a long-term and positive result. This is the advantage in today's healthcare system of going to a Physical Medicine office where multiple providers are all working together on the same patient. Injuries and/or displacements of the spine require special treatment and in the proper sequence to restore the spine's form and function. The role of water intake, supplements, warm-up stretching exercises, force-over-time traction, and isometric-demand exercises, as well as the use of controlled vibration in modern treatment, cannot be refuted. Individual therapies used by themselves are of little benefit in restoration of spinal soft- and hard-tissue form and function in the spinal screw matrix closed kinetic system. Therefore, understanding and using proven protocols is appealing.

Tragedy in the Operating Room

The importance of using non-invasive correction of spinal form and function before resorting to surgery is evident when considering the following statement from orthopedic surgeons, Anthony DePalma, M.D., and Richard

Rothman, M.D., Ph.D., Professors of Orthopedic Surgery, Jefferson Medical College, Thomas Jefferson University. They state: "No operation in any field of surgery leaves in its wake more human wreckage than surgery on the lumbar discs. The situation becomes even more pathetic in the realization that at the start, in most instances, is a healthy, self-sufficient individual. Many of these patients are subjected to numerous operations, and after each operation the patient is worse."

A randomized trial,[32] published as "Surgical vs Non-Operative Treatment for Lumbar Disc Herniation," states, "Lumbar discectomy is the most common surgical procedure performed for back and leg symptoms in US patients, but the effects of the procedures relative to non-operative care remain controversial."

Value of Muscle Rehabilitation

Before launching directly into proven non-invasive correcting procedures, we will first look briefly at a study on lumbar multifidus muscle changes and the role these muscles take in the processes of spinal displacement, rehabilitation, and correction.

A study of the correlation between magnetic resonance imaging (MRI) changes in the lumbar multifidus muscles and leg pain, reported in The Journal of Clinical Radiology,15 was conducted to investigate the relationships between lumbar multifidus (MF) muscle atrophy and low back pain (LBP), leg pain, and intervertebral disc degeneration. In the assessment of the lumbar spine by MRI, changes in the paraspinal muscles are frequently overlooked.

A retrospective study of 78 patients, aged 17–72, presenting with LBP with or without associated leg pain was undertaken. The MRI images were visually analyzed for signs of lumbar MF muscle atrophy, disc degeneration, and nerve root compression. The clinical history in each case was obtained from case notes and pain-drawing charts.

The results of the study showed that MF muscle atrophy was present in 80% of the patients with LBP. This correlation between MF muscle atrophy and leg pain was found to be significant. However, the relationships between MF muscle atrophy and radiculopathy symptoms, nerve root compression, herniated nucleus pulposus, and number of degenerated discs were statistically not significant.

The study concluded that, when looking for atrophy of MF muscle when assessing MRI images of the lumbar spine, the examination of paraspinal muscles should be considered. This may explain the referred leg pain in the absence of other MRI abnormalities.

Remember, the global spine and spinal unit, rather than segmental displacements, are the real spinal displacement complexes. They cause:
- Nerve root compression.
- Hypo-mobility, especially of the lumbar spine, with eventual hard- and soft-tissue pathology. This leads palpation examiners to believe segments are fixated.
- Change of fast-twitch phasic muscle fibers to slow-twitch, especially of the multifidus muscle on the convex side of the subluxation configuration.
- Atrophy of muscles, especially the multifidus on the concave side of the spinal subluxation configurations.
- Normal spinal motion is coupled; that is, lateral flexion and rotation occur as one motion. The multifidus muscle is both a powerful flexor and rotator of the spine.

Chapter 20

Sport Injuries

Sport Injuries

Your first appointment will be no different from the usual osteopathic consultation and evaluation. You will be asked specific questions related to your sport or even to demonstrate some movements. Your diagnosis and treatment plan will be discussed in the usual way.

Treatment is likely to involve the use of osteopathic techniques within the treatment room combined with a more specific exercise-based program in the studio gym. The aim is to return to full physical activity.

Sport & Exercise Medicine Services

Our spinal rehab technicians are highly experienced in the assessment and treatment of soft tissue injuries, with award winning knowledge of biomechanics, tissue pathology and healing. They carry out a thorough assessment, treatment, and rehabilitation for all musculoskeletal injuries.

For complaints including:
- Overuse injuries and stress fractures
- Muscle tears, tendon and ligament sprains
- Knee, ankle and foot injuries

- Shoulder injuries, tennis/golfer elbow, hand and wrist pain

Chapter 21

Durable Medical Equipment

Durable Medical Equipment

Durable medical equipment used by Advanced Physical Medicine is medical equipment used to aid in a better quality of living for their clients at home.

TENS Unit

The T.E.N.S stands for Transcutaneous Electrical Nerve Stimulation. It is an electronic method of controlling pain. Originally developed in the early 1970's, it has been refined into a more compact unit that is easy to use. It works by delivering mild electrical signals through the skin to underlying nerve fibers to alter the perception of pain.

Tens Garment

A conductive garment used with the Tens Unit to treat a joint or larger site of pain such as the entire lower back region. It is also more conducive to the patient in that the patient can relocate the location of the stimulus without assistance.

Lumbar Sacral Orthotic (LSO)

The lower spine carries all the weight of the head and torso, making it the most common site of back pain. Lumbar braces are widely used for the purpose of safe, immediate pain relief and support that is needed to restore functional mobility.

At Advanced Physical Medicine we offer a LSO brace which has a state-of-the-art tightening mechanism that makes it easy to achieve optimal compression of the lumbar spine. The low-profile fit and its ventilated support system automatically conforms to your body for a comfortable fit.

Ankle Foot Orthotic (AFO)

AFO are used for a variety of reasons including:

- weakness or deformity of foot/ankle that requires stabilization
- inability to heel walk
- increased risk of falls
- symptomatic relief and management of chronic intractable pain
- muscle re-education
- prevention of retardation of diffuse atrophy by causing the patient to ambulate

Dakota Unit (Cervical Traction Equipment)

Uses for this device include: Muscle spasms, Pinched nerves, Herniated discs, Fibromyalgia, Spondylitis, Radiculopathy and

Narrowing foramen. The unique design of this comfortable and easy to use cervical traction/stretch device elongates neck muscles and separates cervical vertebrae, often resulting in rapid and prolonged relief from the soreness and irritation that accompanies cervical (neck) problems.

Gentle, intermittent traction exercises the neck muscles increasing circulation. Firm, static traction lowers the pressure between vertebrae, freeing pinched nerves and easing herniated discs.

Chapter 22

Food and Chemical Sensitivity Testing

Food & Chemical Sensitivity Testing

Are Foods Making You Sick?

"Let Food Be Thy Medicine"

Diet plays a critical role in how our bodies function. Every compound that we put in our body is broken down into smaller parts that directly affect and act on our tissues, organs, and larger organ systems.

However, a food item that may give energy and sustenance to one, may cause inflammation and dysfunction in another. Foods, preservatives, and all other digested compounds can cause allergic activation and/or inflammation leading to chronic activation of the immune system. While some may experience significant symptoms, others may have vague symptoms (i.e. fatigue) or none at all; however, these reactions still cause problems within the body.

A few conditions that have been linked to diet and inflammation are:

Migraines, Obesity, Hypertension, Chronic Fatigue Syndrome, Attention Deficit Disorder, Skin Disorders (i.e. Eczema), Digestive Disorders (i.e. Irritable Bowel Disease),

Muscle Aches/Joint Pain, Arthritis, and potentially many more!

Cell Science Systems

The ALCAT Test is now considered the, "gold standard" laboratory method for identification of non-IgE mediated reactions to over 400 different foods, chemicals, and other categories of substances. It is a functional response test and captures the final common pathway of many of the pathogenic mechanisms, immunologic, toxic, and pharmacologic that underlie non-IgE mediated reactions to foods and chemicals. Alcat Test frequently reveals clinically significant reactions that don't fall within the conventional definition of allergy.

This is a test we are offering that measures personalized nutrition at the cellular level. With just one blood draw, this technology will identify foods and compounds that are non-reactive (safe), minimally reactive (OK in moderation), or reactive (harmful). Each plan is highly individualized and will test you for 320 foods, additives, colorings, herbs, preservatives, molds, chemicals (environmental), and 20 commonly used prescription and over the counter medicines.

ALCAT will then customize an individualized nutritional plan and help optimize your wellness by choosing foods that are right for you!

Chapter 23

Vitamin B12

Vitamin B12 Injections can make you again your energy again

Sick of Feeling Sick and Tired?

According to a study (Framingham Offspring Study) more than 39% of 3,000 volunteers had plasma B12 levels in the low normal range. Which for many people can be harmful, yet often goes untreated? "Low normal" is frequently considered 'normal' and overlooked by health professionals. Blood levels are not always the right way to determine whether one needs to supplement, symptoms are better.

Vitamin B12, also called cobalamin is an important vitamin for good health. It can be found in foods such as meat, fish, and dairy products. It can also be made in a laboratory.

Vitamin B12 is required for the proper function and development of the brain, nerves, blood cells, and many other parts of the body. B12 injections have been used for many years by famous personalities and politicians. There are several reasons why:

The injectable route contains 500 times more B12 than the recommended daily allowance.

When injected it is easily absorbed by the body and utilized to form red blood cells and it aids in the maintenance of a healthy nervous and cardiovascular system.

The three primary benefits of vitamin B12 are increased energy (which aids in weight loss), improved sleep, and a feeling of alertness.

Vitamin B12 is also used for memory loss; Alzheimer's disease; boosting mood, energy, concentration, and the immune system; and slowing aging. It is also used for heart disease, lowering high homocysteine levels (which may contribute to heart disease), male infertility, diabetes, sleep disorders, depression, mental disorders, weak bones (osteoporosis), swollen tendons, AIDS, inflammatory bowel disease, asthma, allergies, a skin disease called vitiligo, preventing cervical and other cancers, and skin infections.

Some people use vitamin B12 for amyotrophic lateral sclerosis (Lou Gehrig's disease), multiple sclerosis, preventing the eye disease age-related macular degeneration

(AMD), Lyme disease and gum disease. It is also used for ringing in the ears, bleeding, liver, and kidney disease, and for protection against the poisons and allergens in tobacco smoke.

www.ingramcontent.com/pod-product-compliance
Lightning Source LLC
Chambersburg PA
CBHW070243220526
45465CB00004B/1500